Herbal Therapy:
20 Essential DIY Herbal Remedies and Medicinal Herbs for Fast Use and Natural Healing

Table of content

Introduction

It is well known that food is health care; a medicine is not health care as it is just a cure. In order to enjoy your life at fullest, it is important to be healthy both - physically and mentally. But, if you are suffering from an ailment, then, what would you do? Obviously, you will consult a doctor and rely on pills prescribed by him. But, do you think that the negative side effects of these pharmaceutical pills catch up on you, sooner or later? So, we should check for some natural ways of healing the ailments.

Herbal medicine also termed as phytomedicine or botanical medicine, talk about using a plant's roots, seeds, bark, berries, leaves or flower for healing purposes. Herbalism has an extensive practice of being used as conventional medicine. It is becoming more conventional as enhancements in quality control and analysis, along with improvements in clinical research has revealed the importance of herbal medication in preventing and curing diseases.

During the 19th century, when the process of chemical analysis was known, scientists started extracting and transforming ingredients from plants which can play an active role in treating a certain ailment. Later on, they began creating their own plant compounds, and with a passage of time, drug got more popularity and the decline of herbal medication was started at that time.

This modern era is also moving back towards the herbal medication era, where every disease was cured by the herbal plants. According to some studies about 80% of the African and Asian countries are using herbal treatment as basic medical necessities. There are many factors which result in these statistics. One of them is cost; pharmaceutical medicines are very expensive as compared to herbal medicines. Another factor is easy availability; you can get herbal medicines without any prescription from your doctor.

Other than this, you can easily grow these herbs in your home garden, in this book a list of all the herbs with their usage are given in different chapter and a complete list in tabular form is also given.

These herbal medications have little or no side effects. Sometimes, these side effects may be due to lack of understanding a particular herb or taking the inappropriate dosage. There are different kinds of herbs; some can be used orally while others for external use only. One herb can be used for more than 100 purposes.

Basically, herbal medicines are used to treat conditions like asthma, rheumatoid arthritis, allergies, premenstrual syndrome, migraine, chronic fatigue, fibromyalgia, cancer, and irritable bowel syndrome etc. But as the little knowledge is a dangerous thing so before trying anything consult a doctor or get the guidance of an herbalist. If you are using pharmaceutical medication for a particular ailment then don't use herbal remedies side by side. It may worsen your situation if the compounds in traditional and natural medicines react in a negative way.

So always consult the doctor before using anything, as the health care provider take into account different factors before recommending a particular herb.

Just like the head and tail of a coin, everything has 2 sides, positive and negative. Along with a number of benefits associated with herbal medicines, some side effects are also there. If used properly, herbal medicines can help to treat a range of disorders, but in some cases, may have few side effects. Don't assume them to be safe only because they are "Natural". In certain medical illnesses, few herbs may be unsuitable for people. Herbal medicines are unregulated and mislabeled and often contain contaminants and additives that are not mentioned on the label of medicine. Some herbs may intermingle with pharmaceutical drugs and cause allergic reactions. On other hand, many other herbal medicines are toxic if consumed in high amount or used improperly.

You can learn more about herbs in this book and can easily grow them in your garden; you can even buy few herbs from the market which can be used in food as well as for treatment. An example of such herb is turmeric, it is used in food to make it looks good and taste well. Beside this, it is an anti-bacterial agent and can be used for healing wounds and infections caused due to injury.

Take a look at each chapter and start getting knowledge about different herbs and their usage. I hope this book would help you in creating your home clinic in your garden and in your kitchen cabinets as well, enjoy reading!

Chapter 01: Overview and Benefits of Herbal Medication

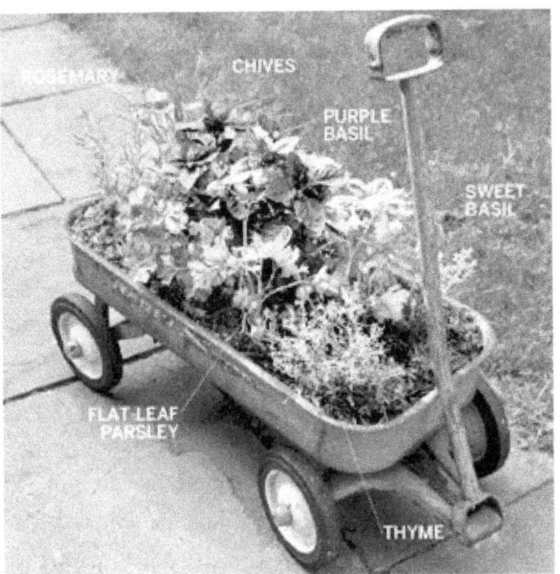

From traditional Chinese medicine to Ayurveda, every medicinal system has made use of herbs for healing purposes. Every herb has more than 1000 uses, some are being used in traditional medicines and some are used in natural ways for treating illness. Herbs are prescribed as they have a tendency to restore the natural balance of the body in a natural way without any side effects.

Herbal medicines are different from the dietary supplement, so both of these should not be confused. Although, they have some components in common, there should be a variance in their usage and their effects on body Nutritional or dietary supplements, do not essentially contain herbal components and are used for adding nutrients to our bodies like amino acid, vitamins, and others. On the other hand, herbal medicine also known as botanical medicine comprises the use of plants for curing purposes.

Everything has its pros and cons, in a similar manner, there are some odds and evens which are associated with herbal medicines. You should consult a naturopath or qualified herbalist before treating yourself with herbs. Always consider the advantages and disadvantages associated with that particular remedy or treatment.

Advantages associated with herbal medication:

Herbal medication is far better than traditional or pharmaceutical medication. If we compare herbal medicines with pharmaceutical medication, then there are a lot of benefits or advantages which we can found in herbal medicines. The benefits are numerous, but some of them are discussed here in detail:

- **Lowers the possibility of side effects:** With the exception of few involuntary reactions, many patients can easily endure and consume most of the herbal medicines as compared to pharmaceutical drugs. It is innocuous to make use of herbal medication over time as they have very rare side effects than those of traditional pharmaceutical drugs. But still consult your doctor or herbalist before taking any herbal medicine as these herbal medicines are unregulated and are without proper dosage information.

- **Operational with chronic illnesses:** You may hear of many long-lasting and enduring health problems that don't retort and react properly to traditional pharmaceutical medicines. In this case, herbal medication has a tendency to be more operational and effective. One such example is the treatment of arthritis with herbs and other alternative therapies.

One of the prescriptions used to treat arthritis, known as Vioxx, was educed due to its negative effects of increasing cardiovascular complications. Beside this, alternating cure results in few side effects, such as dietary changes like excluding vegetables from the nightshade family, the addition of simple herbs and decreasing the intake of white sugar.

- **Herbal medicines are inexpensive:** Herbal medicines are also at an advantage due to cost factor as well. If we compare the cost of prescription medicines with herbs then herbs are less costly and inexpensive. The reasons behind the high cost of prescription medicine are:

- Research

- Testing

- Marketing

So herbs are relatively inexpensive than those of pharmaceutical drugs.

- **Extensive accessibility:** Another advantage associated with herbal medication is that herbs are easily available. You can get them without any prescription from the doctor. At home, some of the simple herbs can easily be nurtured like chamomile and peppermint. In some far-flung areas of the world, the only treatment available for people is herbs.

- **Controls obesity naturally:** As we all know that these days the problem of obesity is on the rise. It leaves dangerous impacts on a person's health. Through herbal medication, this problem of obesity can be controlled efficiently and effectively without making much effort.

- **Natural:** These natural products of the world, herbal medicines syndicate with the immune system to produce a strong detoxification process. According to the principles of eastern medicine, there should be coordination between body and mind, and the superb way to create such a state is to remain in the boundaries of nature.

Although in pharmaceutical drugs the lead compounds tend to be natural, but most often they are combined with artificial and synthetic variables which can result in negative effects.

- **Continued benefits:** To increase the effectiveness of herbal remedy, special instructions about rest, diet, and exercises are given. In this way, our body will respond to the treatment in most desirable and effective way. These lifestyle and dietary changes eventually benefit the patient by bringing their bodies into a healthy tempo. In this way, chances of occurrence of the same illness in future are reduced greatly because these lifestyle changes eventually become a habit and are being followed even after retrieval from that illness.

Chapter 02: Medicinal Plants and Their Uses

Natural plants can have a great healing effect but, we often underestimate it by taking it too lightly. According to the National Park service, at least 175 different plants and herbs are being available for medicinal purposes in the USA. Furthermore, around 60 million people are utilizing herbal remedies in the USA. Now, they are making efforts to harvest these plants from different wild sources. In this chapter, I'm going to share information about 5 common medicinal herbs and their usage.

Ginseng

The location of this herb is Eastern Hardwood forests and total time to reach maturity for this herb is five years. This structure of this plant involves light green flowers, red berries, and green leaves. This plant is used broadly as a medicinal herb because it is good for stimulating our immune system and also results in boosting energy levels. It is also effective if used for lowering the cholesterol and blood sugar level.

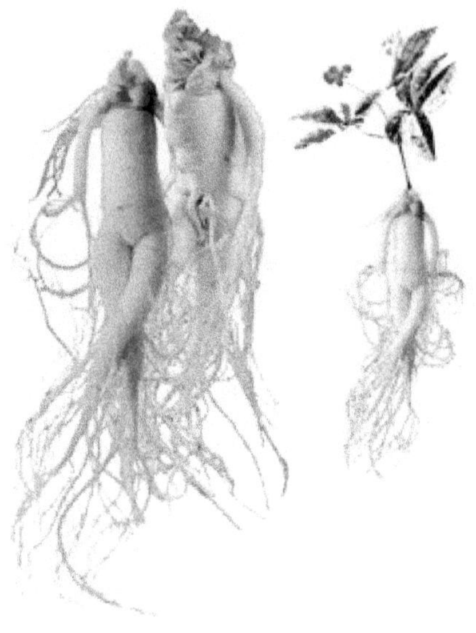

Echinacea

Echinacea plants are resistance to famine or drought so they are stereotypically and naturally found in prairies. Structure includes a large upward pointing bulb, coneflower shape and purple color, small sized petals pointing downward. This herbal medicine is mostly used to strengthen the immune system of our body. Other uses of this plant are to cure:

- Stings and bites

- Burns

- Sores

- Wounds

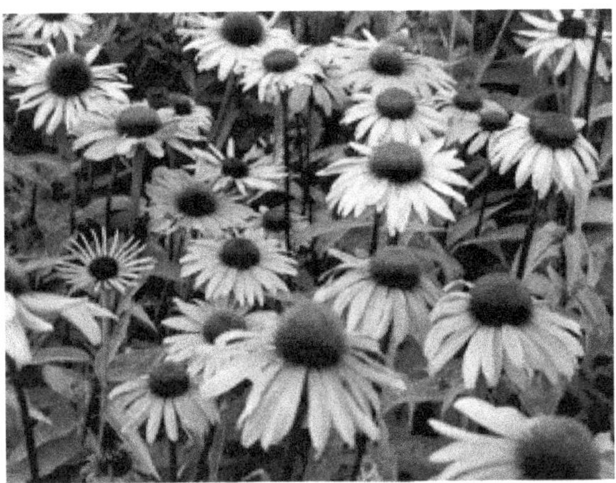

Bloodroot

Bloodroot plant mostly grows in Eastern Woodlands, where it is also termed as "Redroot". You can find it near Solomon's seal or mayapple. Its leaves are round and green in color. Petals are very small and are of white color. The part of Bloodroot plant which is used as medicine is the root. It has the capability to prevent gingivitis and reduce plaque, due to this reason; it has been used as a component in different toothpastes and mouthwashes for many years. Recently, scientists are conducting researches to check whether this bloodroot can be used to cure cancer. In past, it has also been used to decrease the size of tumors.

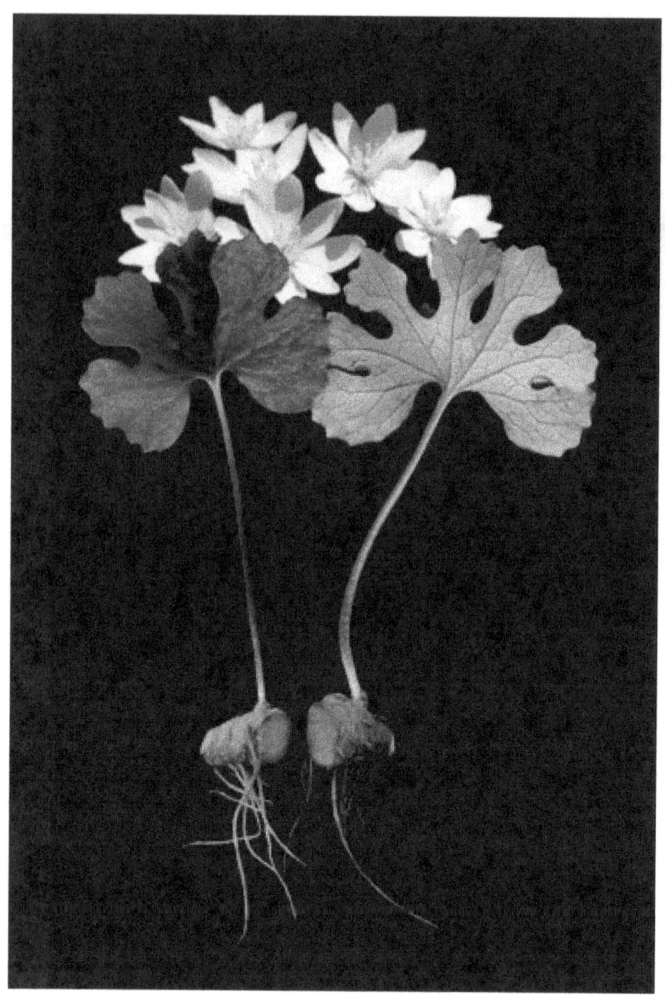

Milk Thistle

Milk Thistle is commonly found in the Mediterranean climates. It consists of a dense flower, tall stem, and small purple color petals. The most common use of this plant is to cure liver as it helps to defend the liver from any harm caused by excessive use of alcohol. Other uses of this plant involve the treatment of:

- Cirrhosis

- Gallbladder

- Hepatitis

Researchers found that this herb is also beneficial for treating patients suffering from depression.

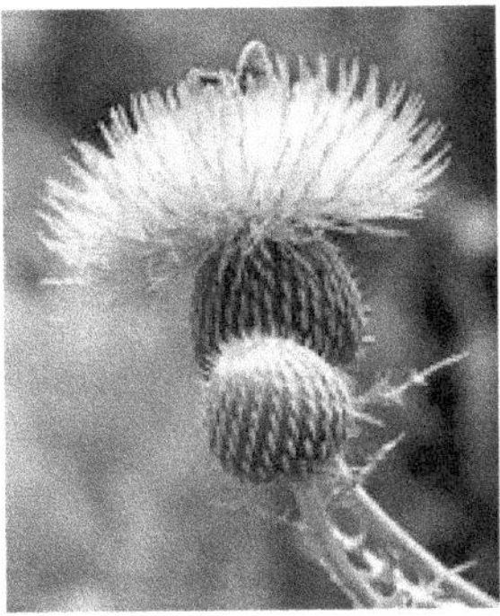

Sage

An exceptional plant known as sage can grow in places with no or little soil, such as dry banks and stony areas. The structure of this shrub includes thin and long leaves of green color with a very delicate flower with purple color petals. For centuries, it has been used as a remedy to cure digestive problems. Other uses of this plant include:

- Healing gum infections

- Healing sore throats

- Profuse perspiration

- Preventing excessive salivation

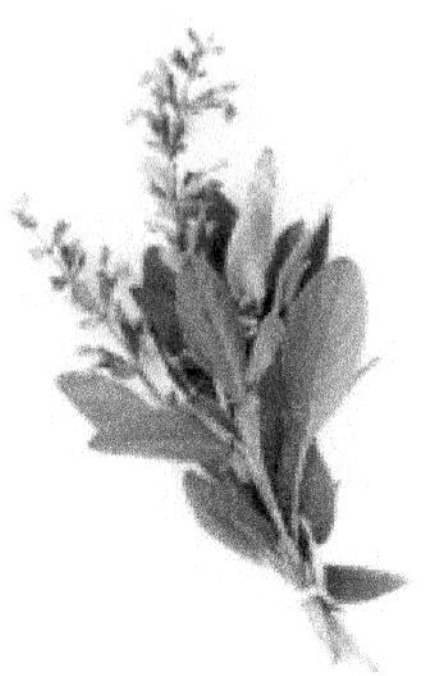

Although these herbs have no or very little side effects, but still remember to pursue the recommendation of a doctor before treating any illness with medicinal plants. In certain situation, excessive use of these medicinal herbs can be deadly.

Chapter 03: Herbal Remedies for Pain, Inflammation, and Aches

Your body can throw your health for a loop at any point in time. Some of the examples are:

- You get grumbling indigestion after eating a seafood-salad sandwich.

- You have an important presentation but you wake up with a sore throat.

- Due to extra workout at the gym, you get back home with a stiff neck.

What if you have a live-in therapist, doctor or trainer to tend to your daily pains and aches? Wouldn't it be great?

Here it goes: recommended by experts, all-natural methods to cure your ailments safely, quickly and effectually at your home. So, clear some area or space in your kitchen cabinet or refrigerator for these amazingly effective and inexpensive herbal remedies. Following are the 10 best home remedies that are similar to have a doctor at your 24-hours service for curing pain, inflammation, and aches

Quell Nausea:

To treat Nausea, the first step is to pervade fresh ginger in water (hot water). Rinse it and then put this mixture in ice cube trays and then freeze. This is known as frozen ginger chips.

When the cubes get frozen then crush them and slurp this icy ginger chips all over the day to deliver a stable and balanced comforting dribble to your tummy. This anti-nausea property of ginger is mainly functional after surgery or during pregnancy period.

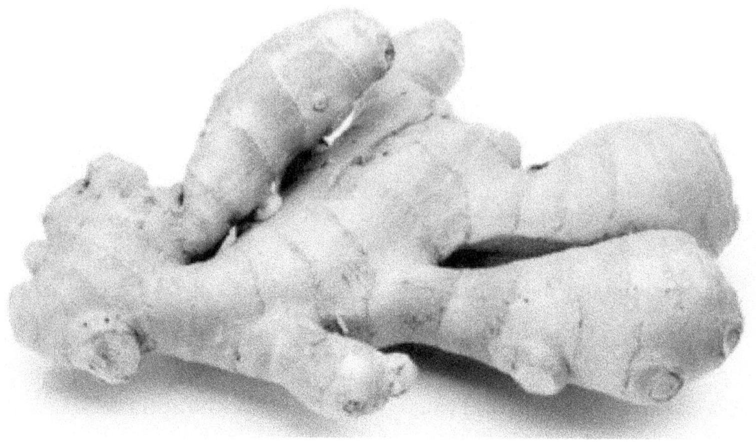

Relax a Sore Throat:

Press six cloves of garlic and mix them in a glass of warm water to make a solution. Use it as a mouthwash and gargle with it daily 2 or 3 times. Repeat this procedure for 3 days. It has been proved scientifically, that there are antimicrobial properties in garlic juice that kill bacteria causing pain in our stomach. The reason for making the warm solution is that this warm garlic juice soothes and calms the inflamed tissues.

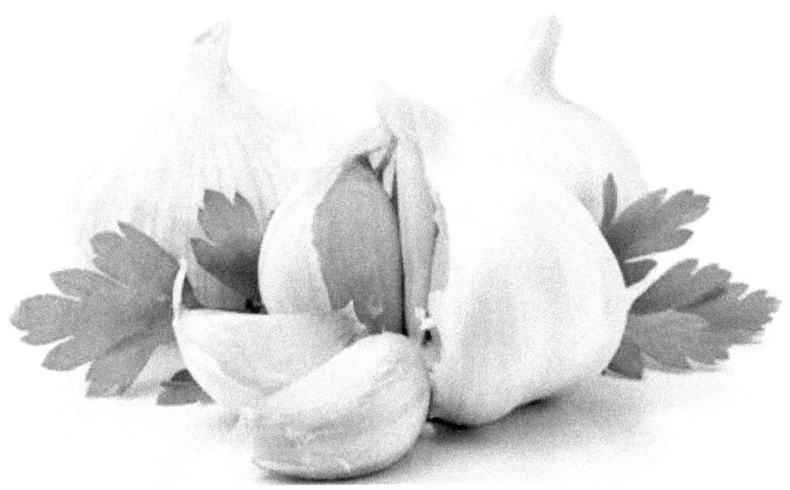

Reduce your fever

If you are suffering from fever, then linden flower tea is a good herbal remedy for you. It functions in two ways:

- It expands blood vessels which induce sweating.

- It helps in stimulating the hypothalamus to regulate your temperature in a better way.

Take 1 tablespoon of linden flower tea and mix it with hot water (1 cup) for about 15 to 20 minutes. Then sip that mixture 3 to 4 times daily. It would help in reducing the fever.

If you are having very high fever, say above 102°F, then take a bath with warm water, it cools your body temperature to become equal to the temperature of water. Continue bathing until your body temperature decreases below 101°F, and then sip a cup of linden flower tea. It would further reduce your body temperature.

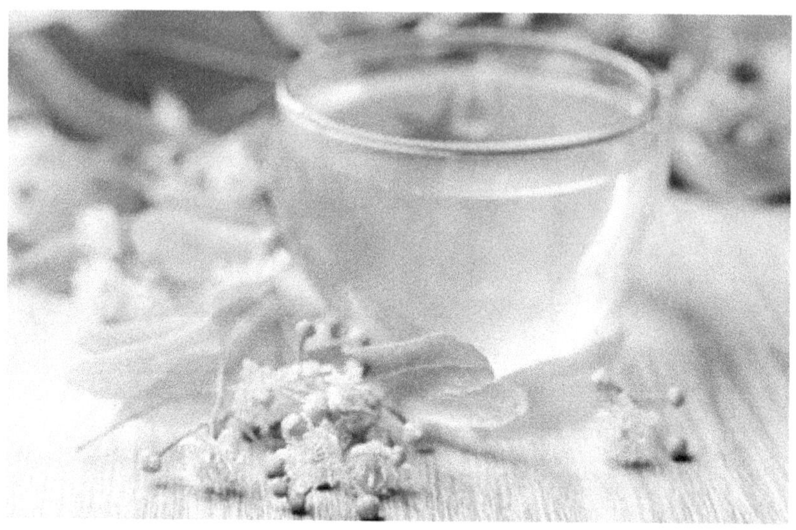

Silent your gassiness:

If you are facing flatulence problem, then use peppermint three times a day. The benefit of using peppermint is that it kills the bacteria that are causing swelling in the stomach. It helps in soothing gastrointestinal muscles for spasm-free and smoother digestion. When you take peppermint, it goes lower in the gastrointestinal tract to start its working. This is the place where gas-plagued individuals require it the most.

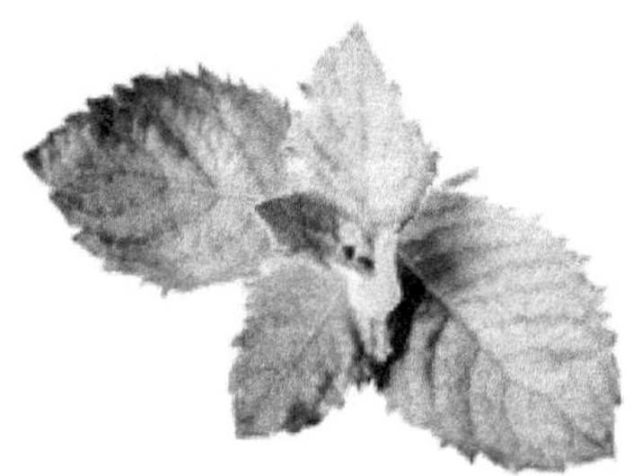

Cut your cold fever short:

Drink faux hot toddy for lowering your high fever. Take half lemon slice and squeeze it in one cup boiling water. Also, drop that half lemon shell into that cup. Also add 1 teaspoon of organic honey; it acts as immunity booster that also cures damaged throat tissues. According to studies, vitamin C is very helpful in shortening the time span and severity of cold. Breathe in the vapors to open the sinuses and to fight the bug drink a cupful 2 or 3 times a day.

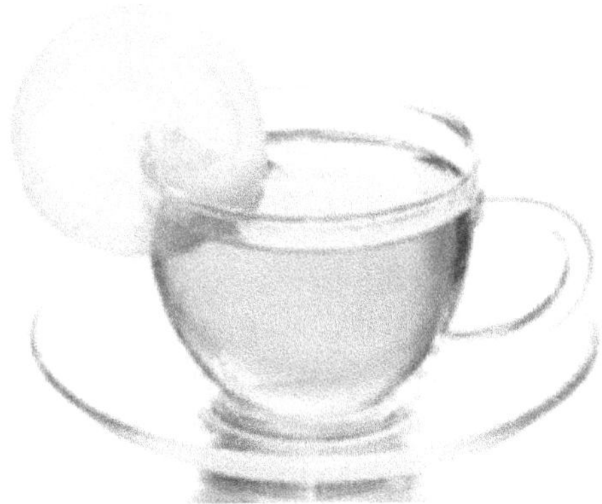

Beat insomnia:

Our body is creating a hormone known as melatonin which is performing the function of regulating sleep patterns. If our body decreases the production of this hormone then it results in insomnia. Scientist discovered that Cherries are jam-packed with this hormone, so before going to sleep, eat a handful of cherries or drink cherry juice. After that, take a bath with hot water to relax your mind and muscles.

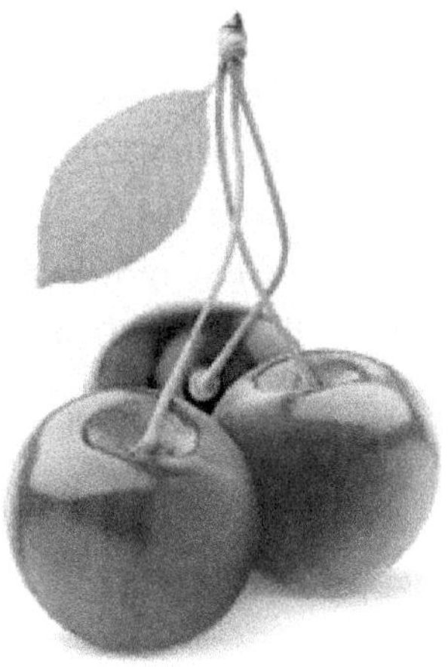

Whiten stained teeth

Things you need for this are; scrubbing pulp of crushed strawberries, a pinch of stain-removing baking soda and water in required quantity to make a paste. Take a soft bristled toothbrush, apply this mixture on it and polish your teeth for few minutes. Repeat this procedure once after every 3 to months. The reason for this gap is that if you do this frequently then it can erode your tooth enamel.

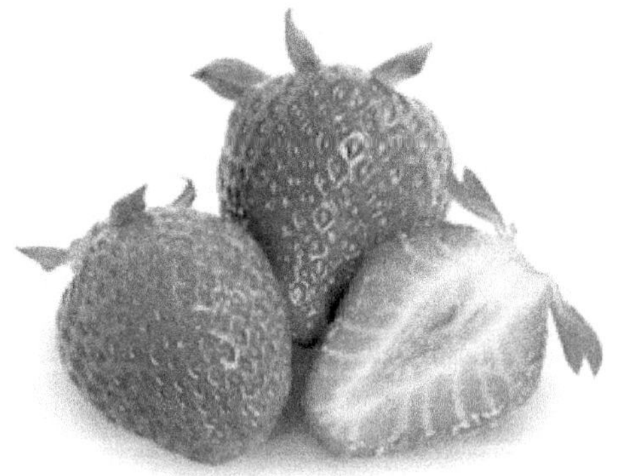

White willow bark

Salicin is the active ingredient in white willow or Salix Alba and our body converts Salicin into salicylic acid. The Bark of this tree helps in lowering the prostaglandins level in our bodies which is a hormone that results in pain, aches and inflammation. Unlike other aspirins, it doesn't cause internal bleeding and upset of stomach. You can utilize this herb for curing following:

* Arthritis

* Menstrual cramps

* Muscle pains

* Hip surgery as it helps in reducing swelling and stimulates blood flow

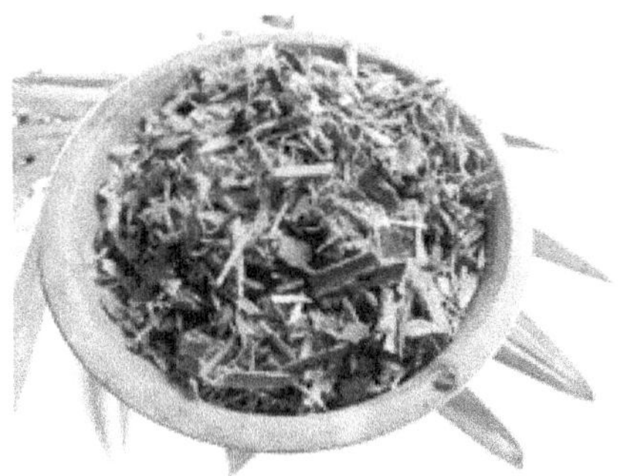

Turmeric:

This is one of the best herbs used to reduce heartburn, inflammation, and to get rid of arthritis. The working mechanism of turmeric against inflammation or pain is still not clear, but this is occurring may be due to Curcumin. Curcumin contains anti-inflammatory characteristics. Although Turmeric is easy and safe to use but as an excess of everything is dangerous, high doses of it can also cause indigestion. Those who are suffering from gallbladder ailment should avoid consuming turmeric.

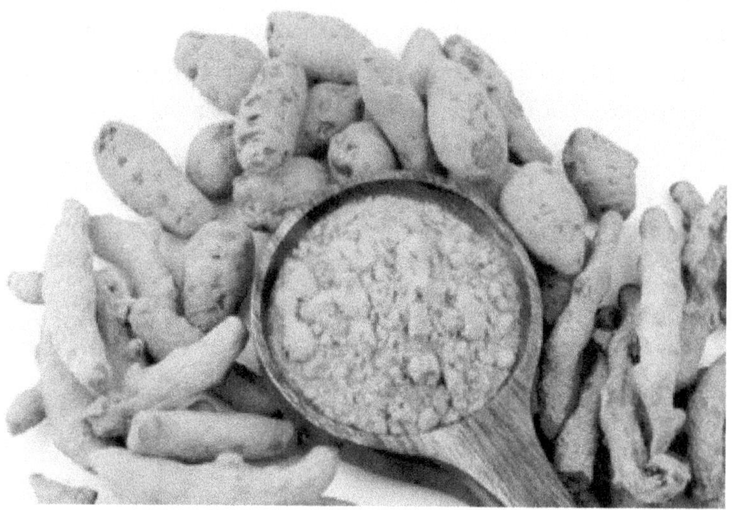

Feverfew:

From centuries, this herb has been used for curing stomachaches, headaches, and toothaches. In modern days, it is also used for rheumatoid, migraines and arthritis. There are no serious side effects linked with this herb, more studies are conducted to endorse whether this herb feverfew is really effective or not. Only a few mild side effects are found which involve irritation of lips and tongue and canker sores. Those women who are pregnant should sidestep from using this

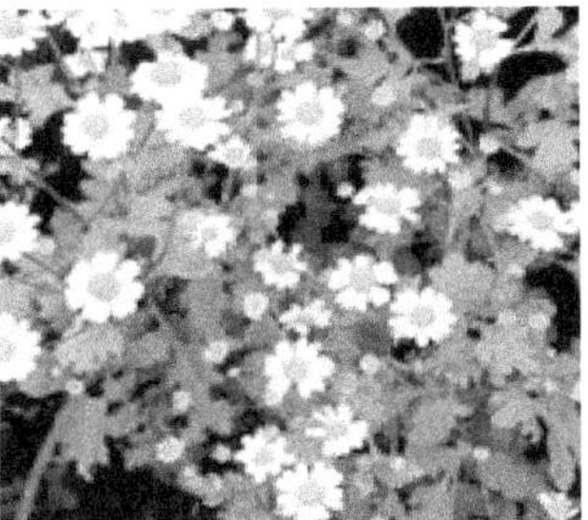

herb as a remedy.

Capsaicin:

Topical capsaicin, derived from hot chili peppers, may be beneficial for some individuals in getting rid of the pain. The working of Capsaicin depends on a substance P, which is a compound that carries the sensation of pain from peripheral to CNS (central nervous system). This depletion of substance P by capsaicin takes few days to occur.

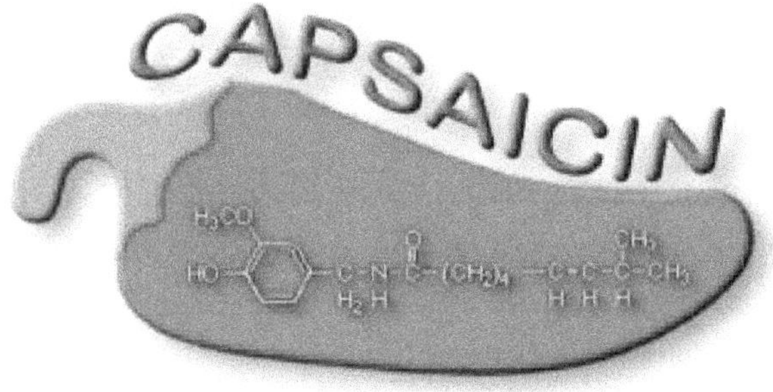

Chapter 04: Herbal Remedies to Boost Immune System and Energy

When the weather outside is chilly and rainy, then it means that the flu and cold season is at its peak. So, it is the time now to pull out all the stops in order to keep our loved ones in tiptop shape and good health. Steady visits to the doctor and proper vaccines are, obviously, a necessity. But, when it comes to preventing illness and stopping the cries on a daily basis, most of us move towards our medicine boxes. Yet, there are many natural ways to cure all these ailments. These natural remedies not only help us to feel good but also help in boosting the immune system of our bodies.

Old age individuals are well aware of the fact that physical abilities, dietary needs, and immunity of body itself all change with age. At that age immune system becomes less responsive due to which vaccines come to be ineffective, resulting in infections.

Getting the right nutrients in your diet is the key to boosting your immune system. But, there are various other steps or ways we can adopt at home to stimulate immunity in ourselves. Herbal teas, gentle exercise, and dietary supplements are a part of naturopathy of naturopathic medicine.

Aloe Vera

Aloe vera is used as an herbal remedy for centuries. You can buy it from natural health store nearby or grow an aloe plant at home. Aloe vera can be consumed orally or topically. If the taste of aloe vera is new to you and is not easy to consume, then start it in a small amount and increase gradually. Before consuming any Aloe vera plant check if it passes quality assurance standards or not. Include aloe vera in your healing kit as it is a superb gel of herbal superfoods.

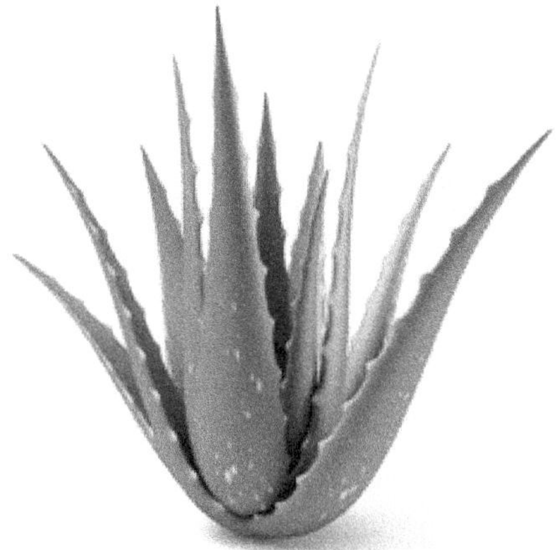

Astragalus:

There are only a few herbal gems in Chinese medicine. Astragalus is one of those herbs that have been used in china for centuries. Due to the healing characteristics of roots of this plant, it is harvested on a large scale. You can buy boiled slices and loose leaves in soups or teas. It is also available in the form of extracts, capsules and powders. It helps in stopping the cold on its way towards you, boost the immune system, and beat the flu as well.

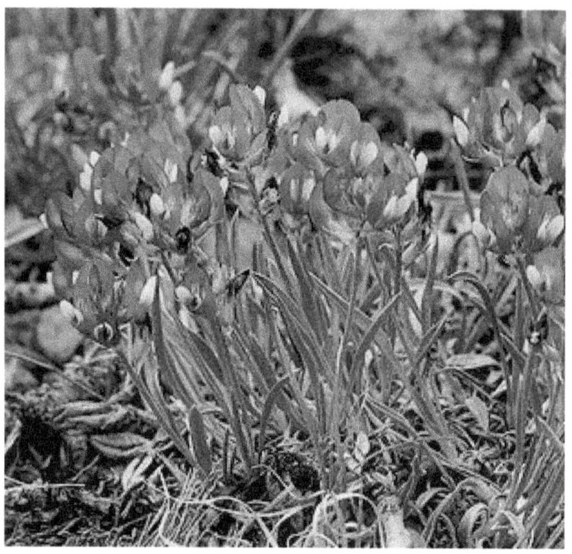

Cat's-claw:

Cat's-claw is enriched with chemicals that boost the immune system to fight against viruses. This medicinal herb acts as a diuretic by stimulating the body to lower blood pressure and lose excess water. According to researchers, cat's-claw can even destroy tumor cell in the body.

Particularly, this herbal medicine is used for treating arthritis pain and aches. You can get relief from rheumatoid arthritis and osteoarthritis due to the anti-inflammatory nature of cat's-claw.

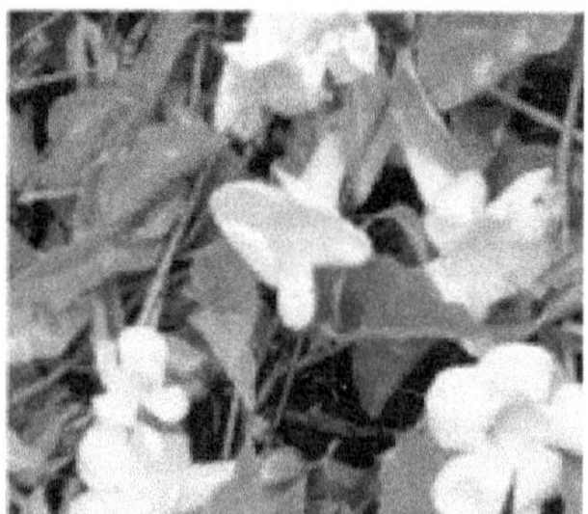

Elderberry:

Elderberry along with some zinc can be the best combination for treating flu and colds. It has great booting antioxidant power due to which it works remarkably to boost the immune system, reduces fever, decreases inflammation, and gives a soothing effect to the respiratory tract.

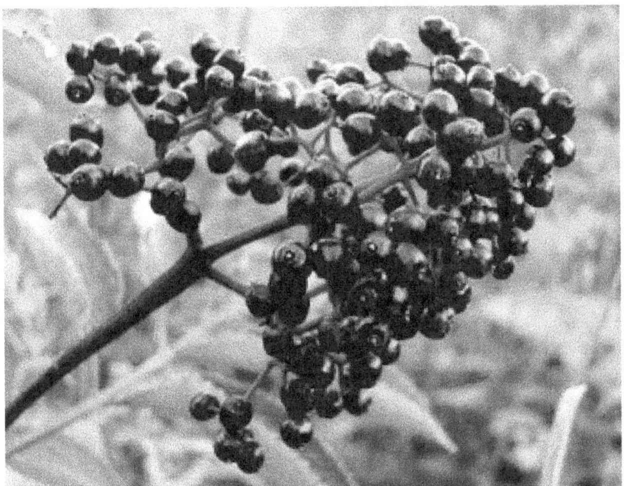

It helps in reducing the severity of the flu and shortens the duration of flu by preventing the flu virus from attaching to the body cells. You can make tincture or sweet elderberry syrup due to its fantastic taste; this is one of the biggest bonuses for elderberry.

1)   Hyssop:

The oil inside the hyssop herb contains healing virtues. This oil contains stimulating effect that arouses expectoration. The major purpose of cultivating hyssop is its flower tops, which are usually soaked in water to make a mixture. This infusion is used as an expectorant to make the mucus loose or thin.

Some other healings by hyssop include arthritis, asthma and wound healing. It is also easily available in the form of capsules, dried herb, tablet, tea or tincture. As it arranges for a catalyst that makes the mucus thin, so the best way to use it is with warm water such as in the form of tea.

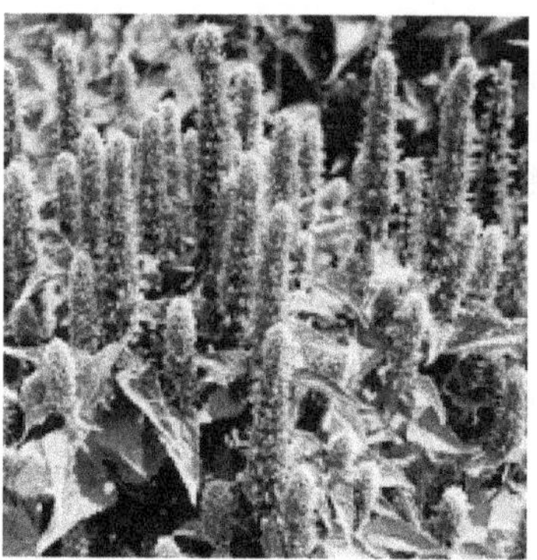

Chapter 05: Common Health Problems and their Herbal Treatments

Now again, pharmacy is moving back to the era of herbal treatment era to bring out and explore benefits for human health. Reasons behind this are the affordability, ease of use and quick healing power to almost every ailment.

Are you interested in growing a small herbal garden of your own as it is fun and benefit for generations? In an emergency situation, your small healing garden would always stance beside you. This chapter is about the most common and important herbal medicinal plants and their usage. Moreover, at the end, a huge list of herbs and their usage is given for you to select herbs for your garden wisely and easily. From the given list, you can easily find out that for a particular ailment what kind of herbs can be used.

Marshmallows:

The roots of this plant are exceptionally advantageous as they cure:

- Bug bites

- Stinging muscles

- bruises and wounds

- Skin irritations

Internally you can treat:

- Stomach acids

- Ulcer

- Urine complications

Chinese Yam:

This Chinese yam can be eaten to treat toxic effects in stomach and spleen. It is also helpful in the treatment of kidneys and lungs. Other cures include:

- Diabetes

- Fatigue

- Dry coughs

- Diarrhea

- Poor ingestion

- Difficulty in urination

- Supports in weight loss

- Scorpio and snake bite

Lemon balm:

The leaves of this plant provide the nurturing appearance and have a mint like smell. It has large flowers, which can be wiped against the skin for:

- Animal bites

- Infections

- Mosquito bites

- Herpes

The nectar is useful for:

- Fevers

- Depression

- Cough and Colds

- Troubled stomach

- Nuisances

- Insomnia

Basil

Have you ever used basil it to cure flatulence? It can also treat:

- Cuts

- Stomach gas

- Lack of appetite

- Scrapes

Tea tree:

Tea tree is famous for curing headache and loss of hair. It comprises amazing benefits like anti-fungal, antibacterial, and works best as antiseptic. In addition to it, it also treats:

- Blisters

- Athlete foot

- Fever

- fatigue syndrome

- Acne and warts

- Vaginal contagions

- Bug bites

Pot Marigold:

This plant can be grown under ordinary climatic circumstances. It is the best herb for treating skin ailments – however, it is also miraculous for external usages like:

- Sore eyes

- Insect bites

- Injuries and stings Ferrari

It also beneficial for curing:

- Infections (chronic)

- Fevers

- Varicose veins

Thyme:

Thyme is famous as a strong antiseptic. It is superb when it is used for the treatment of:

- Stomach gas

- Congestion

- Coughs

Fenugreek seeds:

These are very beneficial and carry excessive nutritional worth – they can cure and treat:

- Labor pain

- Digestion problems

- Drain ducts

- Irritations

- Diabetes (initial)

- Refresh breathe

- Blood cholesterol levels (low)

Turkey Rhubarb

It works best for retaining balance in the digestive system and curing digestion complications. This herb is very placid and cures:

- Constipation

- Bladder problem

- Menstrual problem

- Hemorrhoids

- Diarrhea

Comfrey:

It encompasses allantoin, which helps in replacing damaged cell of the body in a natural way. In addition, it can also cure:

- bronchial problems

- arthritis

- wrecked bones (weak bones)

- severe burns

- sprains

- scratches and acne

- ulcer

Ginseng:

To prolong the life and promote health, this herb is a must to be included in your healing garden. The roots of this herb can be important to treat:

- Nervous disorders (relaxation of nervous system)

- blood pressure levels

- Increase the metabolism rate

- Improve diet

- increased hormone secretion

- Develop immunity

Sage:

Along with curing diseases it can be used in different food items, some of its treatments include:

- Skin infection

- Helps in ingestion

- Gum infection (mouth infections)

- Helps in unclogging menopause

List of ailments and herbs to treat them:

Ailment	Herb
Acne	Calendula, aloe, tea tree
Alcoholism	Evening primrose, kudzu
Allergy	Chamomile
Alzheimer's disease	Ginkgo, rosemary
Angina	Hawthorn, garlic, willow, green tea
Anxiety and stress	Hops, kava, passionflower, valerian, chamomile, lavender
Arteriosclerosis	Garlic
Arthritis	Capsicum, ginger, turmeric, willow, cat's claw, devil's claw
Asthma	Coffee, ephedra, tea
Athlete's foot	Topical tea tree oil
Attention-deficit disorder	Evening primrose oil
Bad breath	Parsley
Boils	Tea tree oil, topical garlic, echinacea, eleutherococcus, ginseng, rhodiola
Bronchitis	Echinacea, pelargonium
Burns	Aloe
Cancer	Bilberry, blackberry, cocoa (dark chocolate), green tea, garlic, ginseng, maitake mushroom, pomegranate, raspberry, reishi mushroom
Cankers	Goldenseal
Colds	Echinacea, andrographis, ginseng, coffee, licorice root (sore throat), tea (nasal and chest congestion)
Congestive heart failure	Hawthorn
Constipation	Apple, psyllium seed, senna
Cough	Eucalyptus
Depression	St. John's wort
Diabetes, Type 2	Garlic, beans (navy, pinto, black, etc.), cinnamon, eleutherococcus, flaxseed, green tea
Diabetic ulcers	Comfrey
Diarrhea	Bilberry, raspberry
Diverticulitis	Peppermint
Dizziness	Ginger, ginkgo
Earache	Echinacea
Eczema	Chamomile, topical borage seed oil, evening primrose oil

Fatigue	Cocoa (dark chocolate), coffee, eleutherococcus, ginseng, rhodiola, tea
Flu	Echinacea, elderberry syrup (also see "Colds")
Gas	Fennel, dill
Giardia	Goldenseal
Gingivitis	Goldenseal, green tea
Hay fever	Stinging nettle, butterbur
Herpes	Topical lemon balm, topical comfrey, echinacea, garlic, ginseng
High blood pressure	Garlic, beans, cocoa (dark chocolate), hawthorn
High blood sugar	Fenugreek
High cholesterol	Apple, cinnamon, cocoa (dark chocolate), evening primrose oil, flaxseed, soy foods, green tea
Hot flashes	Red clover, soy, black cohosh
Impotence	Yohimbe
Indigestion	Chamomile, ginger, peppermint
Infection	Topical tea tree oil, astragalus, echinacea, eleutherococcus, garlic, ginseng, rhodiola
Insomnia	Kava, evening primrose, hops, lemon balm, valerian
Irregular heartbeat	Hawthorn
Irregularity	Senna, psyllium seed
Irritable bowel syndrome	Chamomile, peppermint
Lower back pain	Thymol, carvacrol, white willow bark
Menstrual cramps	Kava, raspberry, chasteberry
Migraine	Feverfew, butterbur
Morning sickness	Ginger
Muscle pain	Capsicum, wintergreen
Nausea	Ginger
Premenstrual syndrome	Chasteberry, evening primrose
Ringing in the ears	Ginkgo
Seasonal affective disorder	St. John's wort
Shingles	Capsicum
Sore throat	Licorice, marshmallow, mullein
Stuffy nose	Echinacea
Tonsillitis	Goldenseal, astragalus, echinacea

Conclusion

This book "Herbal Therapy: 20 Best Medicinal Herbs and Essential DIY Herbal Remedies for Fast Use and Natural Healing" is written with a purpose to provide in-depth knowledge about different herbs and their healing power. I hope you enjoyed while reading this book and now planning to bring some or all of these herbs in your kitchen cabinet, but do one thing before going to buy these herbs. Guess what? Clear some space in your kitchen cabinet or refrigerator!

Although I've provided the detailed introduction about each herb and its usage but still it is requested to consult your doctor before getting indulge in herbal remedies. I each chapter a 5 to 10 herbs are given with all necessary details. While at the end a vast collection of herbs with ailments is given. You can easily check which herb is beneficial for a particular illness. For proper dosage of herbs, please refer to your health care provider as these medicines are unregulated, so no one can tell you the appropriate dosage except the doctor or herbalist.

Thanks again for downloading this book "Herbal Therapy: 20 Best Medicinal Herbs and Essential DIY Herbal Remedies for Fast Use and Natural Healing"; I hope you enjoyed reading this book. Waiting for nice feedback for my book!

FREE Bonus Reminder

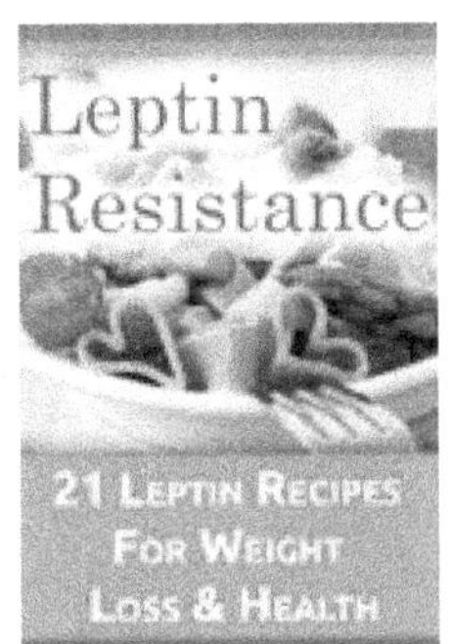

If you have not grabbed it yet, please go ahead and download your special bonus report *"Leptin Resistance. 21 Leptin Recipes For Weight Loss & Healthy Living"*.

Simply Click the Button Below

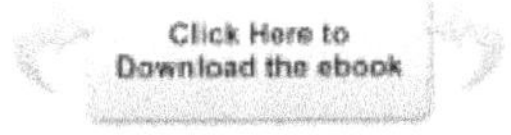

OR **Go to This Page**

http://easyweightlossway.com/free/

BONUS #2: More Free & Discounted Books

Do you want to receive more Free & Discounted Books?

We have a mailing list where we send out our new Books when they go free or with a discount on Kindle. Click on the link below to sign up for Free & Discount Book Promotions.

=> Sign Up for Free & Discount Book Promotions <=

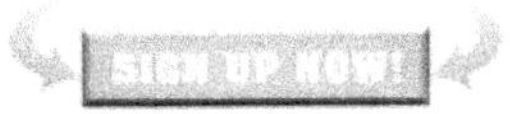

OR Go to this URL

http://zbit.ly/1WBb1Ek

www.ingramcontent.com/pod-product-compliance
Lightning Source LLC
Chambersburg PA
CBHW050802240726
48654CB00008B/597